METABOLIC CONFUSION DIET FOR SENIORS

A Comprehensive Guide Tailored to Enhance Metabolism, Boost Energy Levels, and Promote Optimal Health and Longevity

Dr. Olivia Adams

INTRODUCTION

Welcome to "Metabolic Confusion Diet for Seniors," a comprehensive guide designed to unlock the secret to achieving optimal health, vitality, and longevity in your golden years. Aging is a natural and inevitable part of life, but it doesn't mean we have to settle for diminished well-being, reduced energy levels, or a decline in our quality of life. In fact, with the right knowledge and approach, your senior years can be a time of renewed vigor, improved health, and an enhanced sense of well-being.

In this book, we delve into the powerful concept of metabolic confusion, a dietary strategy that has gained popularity for its remarkable ability to rejuvenate your body and promote positive changes, regardless of your age. It's a concept that challenges the traditional one-size-fits-all approach to nutrition and offers a tailored, age-specific solution for seniors.

Metabolic confusion is rooted in the understanding that our bodies, as they age, undergo a series of physiological changes that require a different nutritional strategy. This approach doesn't just focus on what you eat but also on when you eat, how you eat, and how you move. By harnessing the principles of metabolic confusion, you can revitalize your metabolism, maintain a healthy weight, boost your energy levels, and reduce the risk of age-related health issues.

In this book, we'll explore the science behind metabolic confusion, discuss the unique nutritional needs of seniors, and guide you through creating a personalized meal plan that suits your goals and preferences. You'll find a variety of delicious, nutrient-dense recipes specifically designed for seniors, ensuring that your culinary journey is both enjoyable and healthful.

But our journey doesn't end with nutrition alone. We'll also address common health issues that seniors face, from joint pain to heart health, and provide you with strategies to combat these challenges effectively. In addition, we emphasize the crucial role of physical activity and present age-appropriate exercises and routines to help you stay active and agile.

As you progress through the chapters, you'll discover how to monitor your progress, adjust your dietary plan, and maintain a lifelong commitment to your health. With the guidance of this book, you can take charge of your well-being and age gracefully, embracing your senior years with vitality and confidence.

We understand that every senior is unique, and this book is your compass to navigate the exciting and transformative world of metabolic confusion, tailored to your individual needs and preferences. The journey to better health and well-being starts here, and we're here to accompany you every step of the way.

Are you ready to embark on this transformative journey? Let's dive into the world of metabolic confusion and unlock the path to a healthier, happier, and more vibrant senior life.

TABLE OF CONTENTS

Understanding Metabolic Confusion

1.1 The Science of Metabolic Confusion

Metabolic confusion is a dietary strategy that has gained recognition for its remarkable potential to rejuvenate the body and promote positive changes in weight, energy levels, and overall health. At its core, metabolic confusion leverages the science of human metabolism, utilizing a carefully orchestrated approach to keep the body in a state of adaptability and efficiency. To truly understand the science behind metabolic confusion, it's essential to delve into the key principles that underpin this innovative concept.

1. Metabolism: The Body's Engine

Metabolism is the intricate set of chemical processes that occur within the human body to maintain life. It encompasses everything from converting food into energy to repairing cells and tissues, managing hormones, and regulating body temperature. Our metabolism is influenced by various factors, including age, genetics, diet, and physical activity. As we age, our metabolism tends to slow down, which can lead to weight gain and reduced energy levels.

2. Metabolic Adaptation

One of the central tenets of metabolic confusion is the concept of metabolic adaptation. When we consistently follow a fixed diet or exercise routine, our bodies tend to adapt to the routine, which can lead to a plateau in terms of weight loss and health improvement. Metabolic adaptation occurs when our metabolism becomes more efficient at conserving energy, making it challenging to shed excess weight.

3. The Role of Variability

Metabolic confusion relies on the idea that the human body thrives on variability. By introducing variety into our diet and exercise routines, we can prevent metabolic adaptation. This variety can encompass changes in macronutrient composition, calorie intake, meal timing, and exercise types. When the body encounters change, it has to work harder to adapt, which can lead to increased calorie expenditure and improved metabolic function.

4. Meal Timing and Frequency

In metabolic confusion, meal timing and frequency play a critical role. This approach involves varying the intervals between meals, occasionally incorporating periods of fasting or reducing calorie intake on specific days. By doing so, we stimulate the body's ability to efficiently use stored fat for energy while preserving lean muscle mass.

5. Hormonal Regulation

Hormones are key players in metabolic regulation. Insulin, for example, controls blood sugar levels and can impact fat storage. By strategically manipulating meal timing and composition, we can positively influence insulin sensitivity, which is particularly relevant for individuals dealing with weight management and insulin resistance issues.

6. The Power of Nutrient Cycling

Nutrient cycling is a pivotal component of metabolic confusion. This technique involves rotating different types of nutrients, such as carbohydrates, fats, and proteins, to keep the body guessing. By doing so, we encourage a more balanced utilization of nutrients and avoid the pitfalls of restrictive diets that can lead to deficiencies and imbalances.

7. Continued Adaptation and Results

Metabolic confusion is not a one-size-fits-all solution; it requires ongoing adaptation. As the body becomes more efficient at handling variability, it's crucial to make periodic adjustments to the diet and exercise routines to continue reaping the benefits.

Understanding the science of metabolic confusion is the first step toward harnessing its potential. By embracing variability, meal timing strategies, hormonal regulation, nutrient cycling, and continued adaptation, you can take control of your metabolism, enhance your health, and achieve your weight and fitness goals.

1.2 Why Seniors Need a Specialized Approach

As we journey through life, our nutritional and health needs change, and this transformation is particularly pronounced during our senior years. Seniors face unique challenges and considerations that necessitate a specialized approach to diet and overall well-being. Here, we delve into the reasons why seniors require a tailored and thoughtful strategy to address their distinct needs.

1. Age-Related Physiological Changes

As we age, our bodies undergo various physiological changes. These changes can affect how our bodies metabolize nutrients, respond to exercise, and process medications. For instance, muscle mass tends to decrease with age, which can lead to a decrease in metabolic rate. Bone density may decrease, increasing the risk of fractures. Additionally, the absorption of certain vitamins and minerals, such as vitamin B12 and calcium, can become less efficient. A specialized approach takes into account these age-related changes and offers solutions to mitigate their impact.

2. Nutritional Requirements

Seniors often have different nutritional requirements than younger adults. For example, the need for certain vitamins and minerals, including vitamin D, calcium, and fiber, may increase. On the other hand, the recommended daily calorie intake may decrease as metabolism slows down. Seniors may also need to pay closer attention to factors like hydration and salt intake. A specialized approach addresses these specific nutritional requirements, ensuring that seniors get the nutrients they need for optimal health.

3. Chronic Health Conditions

Seniors are more likely to have chronic health conditions, such as hypertension, diabetes, and osteoarthritis. These conditions often require dietary modifications and careful management. A specialized approach takes these conditions into account, offering strategies to support health and minimize complications.

4. Medication Interactions

Many seniors take multiple medications to manage various health conditions. Some medications can interact with dietary choices, affecting their efficacy or causing side effects. A specialized approach provides guidance on how to manage these interactions and ensure that dietary choices complement the use of medications.

5. Cognitive Health and Mood

Seniors may face cognitive health challenges, including the risk of conditions like Alzheimer's disease and depression. Diet can play a significant role in cognitive health and mood regulation. A specialized approach emphasizes foods that support brain health and emotional well-being.

6. Mobility and Exercise

Maintaining mobility and physical activity is crucial for seniors. A specialized approach to diet and fitness recognizes the importance of age-appropriate exercise and encourages seniors to stay active while considering any physical limitations.

7. Quality of Life

Ultimately, a specialized approach to senior health and nutrition is about enhancing the quality of life. It aims to help seniors maintain independence, vitality, and a sense of well-being. By addressing the unique challenges and needs of this demographic, a tailored approach can contribute to a more fulfilling and active senior life.

Chapter 1: Senior Nutrition Essentials

2. Nutritional Needs of Seniors

2.1 Macronutrients for Aging Gracefully

Aging gracefully is a universal aspiration, and while genetics play a significant role, the food we consume can also influence how we navigate the aging process. Proper nutrition is essential for maintaining good health and well-being as we grow older. The macronutrients—carbohydrates, proteins, and fats—play a crucial role in this endeavor.

Carbohydrates: The Source of Energy
Carbohydrates are the body's principal energy source. They provide glucose, which fuels our cells, including the brain. For seniors, maintaining steady energy levels is vital for daily activities and overall vitality. Choosing complex carbohydrates like whole grains, fruits, and vegetables over simple sugars ensures a sustained energy supply and helps prevent energy crashes. Additionally,

fiber-rich carbohydrates support digestive health, which can become more critical as we age.

Proteins: The Building Blocks

Proteins are the building blocks of the body, and they play an essential role in maintaining and repairing tissues, organs, and muscles. As we age, maintaining muscle mass becomes increasingly important for preserving mobility and overall strength. Adequate protein intake can help with muscle preservation and recovery. Lean sources of protein, such as poultry, fish, beans, and low-fat dairy, are excellent choices for seniors as they provide essential amino acids without excessive saturated fat.

Fats: Essential for Health

Fats have received a mixed reputation over the years, but they are essential for various bodily functions. Healthy fats, such as monounsaturated and polyunsaturated fats found in olive oil, avocados, and fatty fish, support heart health and brain function. Omega-3 fatty acids, in particular, are associated with cognitive health and can help mitigate the risk of age-related cognitive decline. Seniors should aim to include these fats in their diet while being mindful of saturated and trans fats, which can contribute to heart disease.

Hydration: The Often Overlooked Nutrient

While not a macronutrient, proper hydration is vital for aging gracefully. As we age, our sense of thirst may decrease, making it easier to become dehydrated. Dehydration can lead to a range of health issues, including cognitive decline, urinary tract infections, and kidney problems. Hydration promotes good digestion, circulation, and temperature control. Water, herbal teas, and nutrient-rich broths are excellent choices to maintain adequate hydration.

Balancing Macronutrients

Aging gracefully isn't about excluding any of these macronutrients but rather finding a balance that suits your specific needs and goals. A well-rounded diet that includes an appropriate mix of carbohydrates, proteins, and fats, along with sufficient hydration, can help seniors feel more energetic, maintain muscle mass, support cognitive health, and promote overall well-being.

Individualized Nutrition

It's important to remember that individual nutritional needs may vary. Factors such as underlying health conditions, medications, and personal preferences should be taken into account. Consulting with a healthcare provider or registered dietitian can provide guidance on how to customize your diet for optimal health as you age.

Incorporating these macronutrients into your daily diet can be a powerful step toward aging gracefully. By paying attention to the types and amounts of carbohydrates, proteins, fats, and fluids you consume, you can help ensure a healthier, more vibrant journey through your senior years.

2.2 Micronutrients for Senior Health

Micronutrients are essential vitamins and minerals that the body requires in small quantities to support various physiological functions. As we age, paying attention to micronutrient intake becomes increasingly crucial for maintaining good health, preventing age-related diseases, and promoting overall well-being. Here, we explore the key micronutrients that play a vital role in senior health.

Vitamin D: Vitamin D, sometimes known as the sunshine vitamin, is necessary for bone health and immunological function. As seniors tend to spend more time indoors and may have reduced skin synthesis of vitamin D, supplementation or dietary sources become essential. Fatty fish, fortified dairy products, and exposure to natural sunlight are ways to ensure an adequate intake. Maintaining sufficient vitamin D levels can help prevent bone fractures and strengthen the immune system.

Calcium: Strong Bones and More
Calcium is synonymous with strong bones, and it is vital for preventing osteoporosis and fractures. Dairy

products, leafy greens, and fortified plant-based alternatives are rich sources of calcium. As we age, it's essential to monitor calcium intake, ensuring that it's balanced with vitamin D and magnesium for optimal absorption.

Vitamin B12: Cognitive Health

Vitamin B12 is crucial for cognitive function and maintaining healthy nerve cells. Age-related changes in the digestive system can lead to reduced B12 absorption. Seniors should consider fortified cereals, lean meats, and B12 supplements to support brain health and avoid neurological issues associated with deficiency.

Folate (Vitamin B9): Heart Health and Cognitive Function

Folate is important for heart health and cognitive function. It helps regulate homocysteine levels, which can affect cardiovascular health. Seniors should include leafy greens, citrus fruits, and legumes in their diet to ensure an adequate folate intake.

Vitamin C: Immune Support and Collagen Production

Vitamin C is renowned for its immune-boosting properties, and it also supports collagen production, which is essential for skin health and wound healing. Citrus fruits, strawberries, and bell peppers are high in vitamin C.

Vitamin E: Antioxidant Protection
Vitamin E is a potent antioxidant that helps protect cells from free radical damage. Nuts, seeds, and vegetable oils provide good sources of vitamin E, which is essential for skin health and protecting against oxidative stress.

Iron: Oxygen Transport and Energy Production
Iron is critical for transporting oxygen throughout the body and supporting energy production. While iron needs may decrease with age, anemia can still be a concern for some seniors. Lean red meat, poultry, and fortified cereals are iron-rich options.

Potassium: Heart and Muscle Health
Potassium is crucial for heart and muscle health. It helps regulate blood pressure and supports proper muscle function. Potassium is abundant in bananas, potatoes, and leafy greens.

Zinc: Immune Function and Wound Healing

Zinc plays a key role in immune function and wound healing. Seniors can find zinc in lean meats, dairy products, and whole grains.

Magnesium: Muscle and Bone Health

Magnesium is important for muscle and bone health. It supports muscle function and contributes to bone density. Nuts, seeds, and whole grains are rich in magnesium.

Antioxidants: Fighting Cellular Damage

A range of antioxidants, such as selenium, copper, and manganese, help protect cells from oxidative damage. These micronutrients can be obtained from a diverse diet that includes fruits, vegetables, nuts, and whole grains.

Balancing these micronutrients is essential for senior health. It's often best to obtain these nutrients from whole foods, but supplements can be considered when dietary intake is insufficient or when recommended by a healthcare provider. As seniors age, attention to micronutrients becomes increasingly vital to support overall health, maintain cognitive function, and ensure a higher quality of life.

Common Nutritional Challenges

3.1 Digestive Issues

The digestive system is a complicated network of organs that break down food and absorb nutrients. It's a fundamental part of our overall health and well-being. However, as we age, the digestive system can undergo changes that lead to various digestive issues. Understanding these issues and learning how to manage them is crucial for maintaining comfort and good health in your senior years.

Common Digestive Issues for Seniors:

1. Constipation: One of the most prevalent digestive complaints among seniors is constipation. It can result from a combination of factors, including a slower metabolism, reduced physical activity, medication side effects, and dietary choices. To alleviate constipation, consider increasing your fiber intake through fruits, vegetables, and whole grains. Staying well-hydrated and incorporating physical activity into your routine can also help.

2. Indigestion and Heartburn: Seniors are more susceptible to indigestion and heartburn due to changes in the digestive tract and weakened lower esophageal sphincter muscles. Avoiding trigger foods and eating smaller, more frequent meals can reduce the likelihood of these discomforts. If needed, antacids and medications can offer relief.

3. Gastroesophageal Reflux Disease (GERD): GERD is a more severe form of heartburn. It can lead to complications like esophagitis and Barrett's esophagus if left untreated. Seniors experiencing persistent symptoms should seek medical evaluation. Lifestyle changes, dietary adjustments, and medications can help manage GERD.

4. Irritable Bowel Syndrome (IBS): IBS can cause abdominal pain, bloating, and changes in bowel habits. Dietary modifications, stress management, and medication may alleviate IBS symptoms. Consult a healthcare practitioner for specific advice.

5. Diverticulosis and Diverticulitis: Diverticulosis, the presence of small pouches in the colon, is common among seniors. If these pouches become inflamed

(diverticulitis), it can lead to severe abdominal pain. A high-fiber diet can prevent diverticulosis and help manage diverticulitis.

6. Dysphagia: Difficulty swallowing, or dysphagia, can result from age-related changes in the throat muscles. It can lead to choking and malnutrition. It's crucial to consult a healthcare provider for evaluation and recommendations, which may include modified diets or swallowing therapy.

Managing Digestive Issues:

1. Dietary Modifications: Seniors can often manage digestive issues through dietary changes. Increasing fiber intake, staying hydrated, and avoiding trigger foods like spicy or greasy items can help alleviate symptoms.

2. Regular Physical Activity: Physical activity can help to encourage regular bowel motions and relieve constipation. Walking, for example, is a low-impact activity that might be beneficial.

3. Medication and Supplements: In rare circumstances, healthcare practitioners may prescribe drugs or supplements to treat particular digestive difficulties.

4. Stress Reduction: Stress can aggravate stomach issues. Deep breathing, meditation, and yoga are all techniques that can help decrease stress and enhance intestinal comfort.

5. Regular Check-ups: Routine medical check-ups are essential for early detection and management of digestive issues. Seniors should discuss any persistent symptoms or concerns with their healthcare providers.

6. Maintaining a Healthy Weight: Being overweight can contribute to many digestive issues. Managing weight through a balanced diet and exercise is vital for digestive health.

In your senior years, maintaining good digestive health is essential for overall well-being. By understanding common digestive issues and taking proactive steps to manage them, you can enjoy a comfortable and healthy lifestyle as you age. Always seek guidance from healthcare providers for personalized advice and treatment options tailored to your specific needs.

3.2 Dietary Restrictions

Dietary restrictions are a reality for many individuals, whether due to medical conditions, allergies, cultural or religious beliefs, or personal choices. Successfully navigating these restrictions while maintaining a balanced and enjoyable diet can be a challenging but essential aspect of managing one's health and well-being.

Common Types of Dietary Restrictions:

1. Food Allergies: Food allergies can range from mild to severe and may require the complete avoidance of specific foods or ingredients. Common allergens include peanuts, tree nuts, dairy, eggs, soy, and wheat.

2. Celiac Disease: Individuals with celiac disease must strictly avoid gluten-containing grains like wheat, barley, and rye to prevent intestinal damage and associated health issues.

3. Religious or Cultural Dietary Restrictions: Various religious and cultural beliefs dictate specific dietary restrictions. For example, Judaism and Islam have

kosher and halal dietary laws, respectively, which include restrictions on certain types of food and food preparation methods.

4. Vegetarianism and Veganism: Vegetarians exclude meat from their diets, while vegans avoid all animal-derived products, including meat, dairy, and eggs. These dietary choices are often based on ethical, environmental, or health considerations.

5. Medical Conditions: Certain medical conditions, such as diabetes, high blood pressure, and kidney disease, may require dietary restrictions to manage symptoms and maintain health.

6. Weight Management: Many individuals adopt specific diets for weight management purposes, including low-carb, low-fat, or calorie-restricted diets.

Strategies for Navigating Dietary Restrictions:

1. Education and Label Reading: Understanding the ingredients in food products is essential for those with dietary restrictions. Reading food labels and recognizing hidden ingredients is crucial for avoiding allergens and prohibited foods.

2. Substitution and Alternatives: Find suitable substitutes for restricted ingredients. For example, individuals with lactose intolerance can choose lactose-free dairy products or dairy alternatives like almond or soy milk.

3. Meal Planning: Plan meals ahead of time to ensure they adhere to dietary restrictions. This can be especially helpful when dining out or traveling. Carry safe snacks or meals to avoid unintended consumption of restricted foods.

4. Consult with a Healthcare Provider or Dietitian: For individuals with medical conditions or severe allergies, consulting with a healthcare provider or registered dietitian is crucial. They can provide personalized guidance and meal plans.

5. Support and Community: Joining support groups or communities of individuals with similar dietary restrictions can provide valuable advice, recipe ideas, and emotional support.

6. Experiment and Explore: Dietary restrictions need not be limiting. Experimenting with new foods, flavors,

and cooking techniques can lead to exciting and satisfying meals within the confines of restrictions.

Balanced Nutrition with Dietary Restrictions:

It's essential to ensure that dietary restrictions do not lead to nutrient deficiencies. A well-planned diet should provide all necessary nutrients, even with limitations. Nutrient-rich foods, supplements (if recommended), and consultation with healthcare professionals can help maintain a balanced diet.

3.3 Hydration and Senior Health

Staying adequately hydrated is a fundamental aspect of maintaining health and vitality, particularly as we age. The significance of hydration cannot be overstated, and it plays a pivotal role in senior well-being. In this discussion, we delve into the importance of hydration for seniors and how to ensure they receive the proper amount of fluids for optimal health.

Why Hydration Matters for Seniors:

1. Maintaining Organ Function: Adequate hydration is essential for the proper functioning of vital organs, including the heart, kidneys, and liver. It helps in the regulation of body temperature, digestion, and overall metabolic processes.

2. Cognitive Function: Dehydration can impair cognitive function, leading to confusion and difficulties with concentration and memory. Seniors are more susceptible to these effects, making hydration a key factor in preserving mental clarity.

3. Joint Health: Proper hydration can alleviate joint pain and stiffness, a common concern for many seniors. Water helps lubricate the joints and maintain their flexibility.

4. Heart Health: Dehydration can strain the cardiovascular system, potentially leading to an increased heart rate and blood pressure. Maintaining hydration is crucial for overall heart health.

5. Digestive Health: Hydration supports digestion by aiding in the breakdown and absorption of nutrients. It also helps prevent issues like constipation, a common concern for seniors.

6. Skin Health: Proper hydration helps keep the skin supple and may reduce the risk of skin issues, including dryness and itching.

Challenges to Hydration for Seniors:

Several factors can make it more challenging for seniors to stay hydrated:

1. Reduced Thirst Perception: As we age, the body's ability to sense thirst diminishes, making it easier for seniors to become dehydrated without realizing it.

2. Medications: Many medications can have diuretic effects, causing increased urination and fluid loss.

3. Mobility Issues: Limited mobility can make it more difficult for seniors to access fluids, particularly when they're on their own.

4. Cognitive Impairment: Seniors with cognitive conditions may forget to drink or may not recognize their thirst, further complicating the issue.

Strategies for Effective Hydration:

1. Set a Schedule: Encourage regular fluid intake by establishing a routine for drinking water or other hydrating beverages.

2. Monitor Urine Color: Dark urine can be a sign of dehydration. Light, pale urine usually indicates proper hydration.

3. Incorporate Hydrating Foods: Many fruits and vegetables, like watermelon, cucumber, and oranges, have high water content and can contribute to hydration.

4. Use Hydration Aids: Invest in tools like spill-proof water bottles, straws, or cups with handles to make drinking more accessible for seniors with mobility issues.

5. Monitor Medication Effects: Be aware of any medications that may increase fluid loss and adjust fluid intake accordingly.

6. Consider Hydration Apps: There are smartphone apps available that can help seniors track their fluid intake and remind them to drink.

Hydration is a cornerstone of senior health, and it's essential to be proactive in ensuring that seniors receive sufficient fluids daily. By recognizing the importance of hydration, understanding the challenges seniors may face, and implementing practical strategies, we can help our senior loved ones enjoy a higher quality of life in their golden years.

Chapter 2: The Metabolic Confusion Approach

4. Metabolic Confusion Explained

4.1 How Metabolic Confusion Differs for Seniors

Metabolic confusion, an innovative dietary strategy aimed at reviving metabolism and promoting weight loss, is gaining popularity among various age groups. However, the approach for seniors requires specific adjustments to address the unique challenges and considerations they face in their golden years.

Metabolic Confusion Fundamentals:

Metabolic confusion involves the deliberate manipulation of dietary variables to prevent the body from adapting to a fixed routine. The core principles include varying macronutrient composition, calorie intake, meal timing, and exercise routines. These variations force the body to work harder, optimizing calorie expenditure and enhancing metabolic function.

While the fundamental principles remain the same for seniors, there are key differences to consider.

1. Slower Metabolism:

As individuals age, their metabolism naturally slows down. This metabolic slowdown can result in weight gain and reduced energy levels. Seniors may need to adapt their metabolic confusion approach to accommodate these changes by incorporating more frequent exercise, adjusting macronutrient ratios, and paying closer attention to meal timing.

2. Muscle Preservation:

Maintaining muscle mass is of paramount importance for seniors, as it helps preserve mobility and functional independence. The metabolic confusion approach for seniors should prioritize a balanced intake of protein, possibly with a higher protein content, to support muscle preservation and recovery.

3. Nutrient Absorption:

Age-related changes in the digestive system can affect nutrient absorption. Seniors may require dietary modifications, such as increasing fiber intake, to aid digestion and support nutrient absorption. Hydration is also crucial to facilitate nutrient transport and enhance metabolic function.

4. Medical Conditions and Medications:

Seniors are more likely to have underlying medical conditions and take multiple medications. These factors can influence their metabolic function and dietary needs. A metabolic confusion plan tailored for seniors should take into account any medical conditions and potential medication interactions.

5. Hydration and Fluid Balance:

Proper hydration is particularly important for seniors, as dehydration can exacerbate metabolic issues and affect overall health. Seniors should pay special attention to their fluid intake and incorporate hydrating foods and beverages into their metabolic confusion strategy.

6. Cognitive and Emotional Health:

Metabolic confusion can have positive effects on cognitive function and emotional well-being. For seniors, these benefits can be even more significant, given the importance of cognitive health in maintaining independence and quality of life. A tailored approach should consider foods and dietary patterns that support brain health.

7. Joint and Bone Health:

Seniors often face challenges related to joint and bone health. The metabolic confusion approach for seniors should include exercise and dietary strategies to support these areas, with an emphasis on foods rich in calcium and vitamin D for bone strength.

8. Support and Monitoring:

Regular check-ups and consultations with healthcare providers or dietitians are crucial for seniors following a metabolic confusion diet. Monitoring progress, adjusting the approach, and addressing any age-specific concerns are essential for the best results.

4.2 Benefits of Metabolic Confusion

Metabolic confusion is a dynamic dietary strategy that has gained recognition for its potential to promote weight loss, improve metabolic function, and enhance overall well-being. By deliberately introducing variation in your diet and exercise routines, metabolic confusion can deliver a range of benefits that appeal to individuals of various age groups, lifestyles, and health goals. Here are the key advantages of adopting a metabolic confusion approach:

1. Enhanced Weight Loss:

One of the primary benefits of metabolic confusion is its capacity to promote weight loss. By avoiding the plateau effect that often accompanies rigid diet and exercise routines, metabolic confusion keeps the body from adapting to a fixed pattern. This leads to consistent calorie burning and facilitates the shedding of excess pounds, even in stubborn areas.

2. Revitalized Metabolism:

Metabolic confusion encourages your metabolism to remain active and responsive. This adaptive process prevents metabolic slowdown, ensuring that your body continues to efficiently burn calories, even as you age. This is particularly beneficial for seniors who may experience a natural decline in metabolic rate.

3. Improved Insulin Sensitivity:

Metabolic confusion can positively impact insulin sensitivity, which is crucial for blood sugar regulation. By varying meal timing and macronutrient composition, this approach can help stabilize blood sugar levels, reducing the risk of insulin resistance and type 2 diabetes.

4. Muscle Preservation:

The approach of metabolic confusion emphasizes a balanced intake of macronutrients, including protein, to support muscle preservation and recovery. This is particularly advantageous for those looking to maintain lean muscle mass while losing weight or for seniors who wish to preserve mobility and functional independence.

5. Cognitive Benefits:

Studies suggest that metabolic confusion may have positive effects on cognitive function. By supporting brain health and emotional well-being, this dietary approach can help improve focus, memory, and overall mental clarity.

6. Sustainable Weight Maintenance:

Metabolic confusion is not just about losing weight but also about maintaining it over the long term. By fostering a flexible and adaptable metabolism, this approach promotes a sustainable, balanced lifestyle that reduces the likelihood of weight regain.

7. Versatility and Customization:

Metabolic confusion offers flexibility and can be customized to suit individual preferences and goals. Whether you prefer low-carb, high-fat, or balanced diets, metabolic confusion can be adapted to accommodate your specific dietary choices.

8. Nutrient-Rich Diet:

By encouraging the incorporation of a variety of foods, metabolic confusion supports a nutrient-rich diet. This approach helps ensure that you receive a wide array of essential vitamins, minerals, and antioxidants necessary for overall health.

9. Positive Psychological Impact:

Metabolic confusion can be mentally liberating, as it allows for occasional indulgences and flexibility within your dietary plan. This can reduce the feelings of restriction and deprivation commonly associated with traditional diets, promoting a healthier relationship with food.

10. Fitness and Agility:

Exercise routines complement the metabolic confusion approach, supporting your fitness goals and overall agility. The combination of dietary variation and age-appropriate physical activity can keep you active and energetic.

11. Individualized Health Solutions:

Metabolic confusion is adaptable to various age groups, making it a valuable tool for seniors looking to enhance their vitality and health. By understanding age-specific needs and limitations, this approach can be tailored to address the unique challenges faced by older individuals.

Tailoring the Diet for Seniors

5.1 Safety Considerations

While metabolic confusion and similar dietary strategies offer potential benefits, it's essential to approach them with care and consider various safety aspects. Here are some key safety considerations to keep in mind when adopting these dietary approaches:

1. Consult with a Healthcare Provider:

Before embarking on any significant dietary changes, especially if you have underlying medical conditions, it's crucial to consult with a healthcare provider. They can evaluate your specific health status and provide personalized guidance to ensure that the chosen dietary approach is safe and suitable for your individual needs.

2. Address Food Allergies and Sensitivities:

If you have known food allergies or sensitivities, ensure that your chosen dietary approach accommodates these restrictions. Allergen exposure can lead to severe reactions, so careful planning and label reading are essential.

3. Medication and Nutrient Interactions:

Certain dietary strategies can interact with medications, potentially reducing their effectiveness or causing adverse effects. Inform your healthcare provider about any changes to your diet and seek their guidance to ensure that dietary choices do not compromise your medication regimen.

4. Gradual Transition:

Sudden, drastic changes in diet can lead to digestive discomfort, such as bloating, gas, and diarrhea. To minimize these issues, consider a gradual transition into a metabolic confusion or other dietary strategy. Slowly introduce variations to give your body time to adapt.

5. Stay Hydrated:

Metabolic confusion and similar dietary approaches may require alterations in fluid intake. Ensure that you remain adequately hydrated, as dehydration can lead to various health issues, including kidney stones and electrolyte imbalances.

6. Monitoring and Adjustment:

Consistently monitor your progress and well-being. If you experience adverse effects, such as excessive weight loss, fatigue, dizziness, or nutritional deficiencies, consider adjusting your dietary plan accordingly.

7. Nutrient Balance:

Maintaining a balanced diet is essential to avoid nutrient deficiencies. Adequate intake of essential vitamins, minerals, and macronutrients is vital for overall health. Dietary variety and, when necessary, supplementation can help achieve nutrient balance.

8. Listen to Your Body:

Pay attention to your body's signals. If you experience persistent discomfort or negative side effects, it's essential to address them promptly. Avoid pushing your body beyond its limits.

9. Psychological Well-Being:

The psychological aspect of dietary strategies is crucial. Avoid extremes that may lead to unhealthy relationships with food or body image. Dietary approaches should promote overall well-being, including mental health.

10. Adapt for Your Age:

Seniors should take age-specific considerations into account when implementing metabolic confusion. This may include adjustments in exercise intensity, nutrient density, and hydration practices.

11. Monitor Weight Loss:

While weight loss can be a goal for many individuals, excessive and rapid weight loss can be harmful. Ensure that your dietary approach supports gradual and sustainable weight management.

5.2 Meal Timing and Frequency

The timing and frequency of meals play a significant role in our overall health and well-being. How we structure our daily food intake can impact our metabolism, energy levels, and even our weight management. Here's an exploration of the importance of meal timing and frequency in our diets:

1. Balancing Blood Sugar:

Eating at regular intervals helps maintain stable blood sugar levels. This is essential for energy and mood regulation, as blood sugar spikes and crashes can lead to fatigue, irritability, and cravings for unhealthy foods. Aim to consume balanced meals and snacks throughout the day to keep blood sugar levels steady.

2. Metabolic Rate:

Meal frequency can influence our metabolic rate. Regular eating can help keep the metabolism active, as the body needs to expend energy to digest and process food. However, excessively frequent eating can lead to overconsumption of calories, so finding the right balance is key.

3. Appetite Control:

Frequent meals and snacks can help control appetite and prevent overeating. When you eat at regular intervals, you're less likely to experience extreme hunger, which can lead to poor food choices and overindulgence.

4. Nutrient Absorption:

Nutrient absorption can be more efficient when meals are spaced throughout the day. Breaking your daily nutrient intake into multiple meals allows your body to absorb and utilize the nutrients more effectively.

5. Satiety:

Proper meal timing and spacing can enhance the feeling of fullness, making it easier to control portions and reduce the risk of overeating. Eating at regular intervals signals to your body that it's getting nourishment, which can prevent excessive hunger.

6. Weight Management:

Some studies suggest that frequent, smaller meals can support weight management by preventing excessive calorie intake. However, the overall number of calories you consume in a day is still a crucial factor in weight control.

7. Energy Levels:

Optimal meal timing can help maintain steady energy levels throughout the day. Eating a balanced breakfast, for example, kickstarts your metabolism and provides the energy you need to start the day. Regular meals and snacks can help sustain this energy.

8. Dietary Choices:

When you eat at regular intervals, you have more opportunities to make healthier dietary choices. Instead of reaching for convenient, high-calorie snacks, you can plan balanced meals and snacks that align with your nutritional goals.

9. Personalized Approach:

Meal timing and frequency can vary from person to person. Some individuals thrive on three square meals a day, while others may prefer several smaller meals. It's essential to find an eating pattern that suits your lifestyle, appetite, and health goals.

10. Timing Matters:

The timing of your last meal can also affect sleep quality. Eating heavy or spicy foods too close to bedtime can lead to discomfort and disrupted sleep. It's advisable to allow a few hours between your last meal and bedtime.

11. Consistency is Key:

Consistency in meal timing can help regulate your body's internal clock, supporting overall health. Irregular eating patterns can disrupt your circadian rhythms, potentially affecting sleep, digestion, and metabolism.

Chapter 3: Planning Your Senior Metabolic Confusion Diet

Creating a Personalized Meal Plan

6.1 Daily Meal Structure

The daily meal structure plays a pivotal role in shaping our nutritional habits and overall well-being. By establishing a consistent and balanced approach to how we eat, we can support our energy levels, metabolism, and long-term health. Here's a breakdown of an ideal daily meal structure:

1. Breakfast: The Morning Kickstart

Breakfast is often considered the most important meal of the day as it jumpstarts your metabolism and provides energy for the day ahead. A well-rounded breakfast typically includes a source of carbohydrates (like whole grains), protein (such as eggs or yogurt), and healthy fats (like avocado or nuts). This combination helps maintain steady blood sugar levels and keeps you full until your next meal.

2. Mid-Morning Snack: Sustaining Energy

A mid-morning snack can be especially helpful if your breakfast was on the lighter side. Choose a nutritious option like fruit, yogurt, or a handful of nuts to keep your energy levels stable.

3. Lunch: The Midday Sustenance

Lunch is your opportunity to refuel and nourish your body. Include a source of lean protein (such as chicken, tofu, or beans), plenty of vegetables, and complex carbohydrates (like quinoa or brown rice). This combination provides essential nutrients and helps prevent the mid-afternoon energy slump.

4. Afternoon Snack: Keeping Hunger at Bay

An afternoon snack can help you avoid overeating at dinner. Opt for a balanced option, such as a piece of fruit, vegetables with hummus, or a small serving of Greek yogurt.

5. Dinner: A Nutrient-Rich End to the Day

Dinner should include lean protein, vegetables, and a moderate serving of carbohydrates. This combination helps satisfy hunger and provides essential nutrients for recovery and overnight repair.

6. Evening Snack (Optional): Light Fare

An evening snack is optional and should be light. If you're hungry before bedtime, consider a small, healthy option like a piece of fruit or a handful of nuts. Avoid heavy or spicy foods that can disrupt your sleep.

Additional Considerations:

Hydration: Incorporate water, herbal teas, and hydrating foods throughout the day to stay well-hydrated. Adequate hydration supports digestion, energy levels, and overall health.

Portion Control: To avoid overeating, keep portion proportions in mind. Pay attention to hunger cues and eat until you're comfortably satisfied, not overly full.

Meal Timing: Try to eat at consistent intervals each day. This routine helps regulate your body's internal clock and can improve digestion and metabolism.

Variety: Aim for a diverse diet with a wide range of foods to ensure you get a broad spectrum of nutrients. Rotate your choices to keep meals interesting and to meet your nutritional needs.

Personalization: Adapt your daily meal structure to your lifestyle, dietary preferences, and health goals. What works for one person may not work for another, so tailor your approach to your unique needs.

6.2 Food Choices for Seniors

As we age, our dietary needs and food choices evolve, becoming even more crucial to maintain good health, energy, and overall well-being. The right food choices for seniors can support healthy aging, prevent chronic diseases, and enhance quality of life. Here's a guide to making informed and healthful food choices in your senior years:

1. Prioritize Nutrient-Dense Foods:

As we age, our calorie needs may decrease, making it essential to prioritize nutrient-dense foods. Choose foods rich in vitamins, minerals, and antioxidants while limiting empty-calorie options. Opt for fruits, vegetables, whole grains, lean proteins, and healthy fats.

2. Protein for Muscle Health:

Adequate protein intake is vital for maintaining muscle mass and preventing muscle loss, a common issue in seniors. Include sources of lean protein in your diet, such as poultry, fish, lean meats, eggs, beans, and low-fat dairy products.

3. Fiber for Digestive Health:

Fiber is crucial for digestive health and preventing constipation, a common issue in older adults. Incorporate high-fiber foods like whole grains, legumes, fruits, and vegetables into your daily meals.

4. Calcium and Vitamin D for Bone Health:

Maintaining strong bones is essential for seniors to prevent fractures and osteoporosis. Consume dairy products, fortified plant-based milk, leafy greens, and seafood to ensure you get enough calcium. Vitamin D, obtained from sunlight and fortified foods, helps your body absorb calcium.

5. Healthy Fats for Heart Health:

Opt for healthy fats found in foods like avocados, nuts, seeds, and fatty fish (like salmon and trout). These fats support heart health and cognitive function.

6. Hydration Matters:

Seniors are at a higher risk of dehydration, which can lead to various health issues. Be conscious of your fluid intake and include hydrating foods like water-rich fruits and vegetables in your diet.

7. Limit Sodium and Processed Foods:

Excessive sodium intake can lead to high blood pressure and cardiovascular issues. Limit your consumption of processed and packaged foods, which often contain hidden sources of salt.

8. Focus on Whole Foods:

Whole foods are minimally processed and retain their natural nutrients. They should form the foundation of your diet. Choose fresh produce, whole grains, and unprocessed meats.

9. Balance Your Diet:

A well-balanced diet should include a variety of foods from all food groups. Incorporate a rainbow of fruits and vegetables, lean proteins, whole grains, and healthy fats into your meals.

10. Be Mindful of Special Dietary Needs:

Seniors may have specific dietary requirements due to medical conditions. If you have diabetes, heart disease, or other health concerns, work with a healthcare provider or registered dietitian to create a tailored meal plan.

11. Portion Control:

As metabolism naturally slows with age, be mindful of portion sizes. Listen to your body's hunger cues and aim for smaller, balanced meals.

12. Enjoy Social Meals:

Sharing meals with friends and family can enhance your emotional well-being. Social meals provide not only nourishment but also companionship and a sense of connection.

6.3 Sample Meal Plans

Creating a well-balanced meal plan tailored to the nutritional needs of seniors is essential for maintaining health and vitality. Here are some sample meal plans that illustrate how to structure daily meals for optimal nourishment:

Sample Meal Plan 1: Balanced Diet for Seniors

Breakfast:

Scrambled eggs with spinach and tomatoes
Whole-grain toast
Fresh orange slices
Mid-Morning Snack:

Greek yogurt with honey and a sprinkle of nuts
Lunch:

Grilled chicken breast salad with mixed greens, cherry tomatoes, cucumbers, and a vinaigrette dressing
Quinoa or brown rice

Afternoon Snack:

Sliced apples with peanut butter
Dinner:

Baked salmon with lemon and dill
Steamed broccoli
Mashed sweet potatoes
Sample Meal Plan 2: Vegetarian Senior Meal Plan

Breakfast:

Oatmeal topped with berries and chopped nuts
A glass of calcium-fortified plant-based milk
Mid-Morning Snack:

Hummus accompanied by carrot and cucumber sticks

Lunch: lentil soup with whole-grain crackers

Salad of mixed greens with balsamic vinaigrette

Afternoon Snack: Greek yogurt with honey drizzle

Dinner:

Grilled tofu with stir-fried vegetables (bell peppers,
zucchini, and broccoli)
Quinoa or brown rice
Sample Meal Plan 3: Heart-Healthy Senior Meal Plan

Breakfast:

Whole-grain cereal with skim milk
Fresh berries
Mid-Morning Snack:

Handful of almonds
Lunch:

Grilled salmon with a side of steamed asparagus
Quinoa or whole-grain pasta
Afternoon Snack:

Sliced peaches with cottage cheese
Dinner:

Baked chicken breast with a side of roasted Brussels
sprouts
Brown rice

Sample Meal Plan 4: Low-Sodium Senior Meal Plan

Breakfast:

Scrambled egg whites with sautéed spinach
Whole-grain toast
Fresh orange slices
Mid-Morning Snack:

Low-sodium vegetable juice
Lunch:

Grilled turkey sandwich on whole-grain bread with plenty of veggies
A side of low-sodium vegetable soup
Afternoon Snack:

Sliced cucumber and red pepper with hummus
Dinner:

Baked cod with lemon and herbs
Steamed green beans
Quinoa

**Sample Meal Plan 5: Diabetes-Friendly Senior
Meal Plan**

Breakfast:

Overnight oats with almond milk, chia seeds, and
berries
A small apple
Mid-Morning Snack:

Low-fat yogurt with a sprinkle of cinnamon
Lunch:

Grilled chicken breast salad with mixed greens and a
vinaigrette dressing
Quinoa
Afternoon Snack:

Sliced pear with a few almonds
Dinner:

Baked salmon with a lemon-dill sauce
Steamed broccoli
Cauliflower rice

Day 6:

Breakfast:

Scrambled egg whites with sautéed mushrooms and
spinach
Whole-grain toast
A small banana
Mid-Morning Snack:

Low-fat cottage cheese with pineapple chunks
Lunch:

Grilled shrimp and avocado salad with mixed greens
and a lime-cilantro dressing
Quinoa
Afternoon Snack:

Sliced bell peppers with guacamole
Dinner:

Baked chicken breast with a Mediterranean-style
tomato and olive topping
Steamed green beans
Brown rice

Day 7:

Breakfast:

Plain Greek yogurt with honey, walnuts, and a sprinkle of granola
Mixed berries
Mid-Morning Snack:

A handful of cherry tomatoes
Lunch:

Turkey and vegetable stir-fry with a light ginger-soy sauce
Brown rice
Afternoon Snack:

Sliced peaches with a dollop of low-fat whipped cream
Dinner:

Baked cod with a lemon-caper sauce
Steamed asparagus
Quinoa

Remember that these sample meal plans are just a starting point. Seniors should tailor their diets to their unique nutritional needs, dietary preferences, and any medical conditions they may have. Consulting with a healthcare provider or registered dietitian is essential for creating a personalized meal plan that supports individual health and well-being goals.

Chapter 4: Combating Common Senior Health Issues

7. Arthritis and Joint Health

7.1 Foods to Alleviate Joint Pain

Joint pain is a common concern, especially as we age. While medication and physical therapy can be effective treatments, your diet also plays a significant role in managing joint discomfort and promoting joint health. Certain foods are rich in nutrients and compounds that can help alleviate joint pain and inflammation. Here are some of the best options:

1. Fatty Fish:

Fatty fish like salmon, mackerel, sardines, and trout are abundant in omega-3 fatty acids. These essential fats have powerful anti-inflammatory properties that can help reduce joint pain and stiffness. Aim to include fatty fish in your diet at least two times a week.

2. Turmeric:

Turmeric contains curcumin, a potent anti-inflammatory compound. Adding turmeric to your meals or consuming it as a supplement may help alleviate joint pain and inflammation. Consider making turmeric tea or adding it to curries and soups.

3. Ginger:

Ginger is another natural anti-inflammatory spice. It can be added to dishes, used in tea, or consumed as a supplement. Ginger has been shown to reduce symptoms of osteoarthritis and may provide relief from joint pain.

4. Berries:

Berries like strawberries, blueberries, and raspberries are rich in antioxidants, particularly anthocyanins. These compounds help combat inflammation and oxidative stress, potentially reducing joint discomfort.

5. Nuts and Seeds:

Almonds, walnuts, flaxseeds, and chia seeds are excellent sources of healthy fats and antioxidants. These foods can help reduce inflammation and may contribute to joint pain relief.

6. Green Tea:

Green tea contains polyphenols, which have anti-inflammatory properties. Drinking green tea regularly may help manage joint pain and promote overall health.

7. Broccoli:

Broccoli is packed with vitamins, minerals, and a compound called sulforaphane, which has anti-inflammatory effects. Including broccoli in your meals can be beneficial for joint health.

8. Oranges and Citrus Fruits:

Oranges and other citrus fruits are high in vitamin C, which is essential for collagen production. Collagen is a vital component of joint cartilage, and maintaining its health can help alleviate joint pain.

9. Olive Oil:

Extra virgin olive oil is a healthy fat rich in monounsaturated fats and antioxidants. It can help reduce inflammation and may contribute to improved joint comfort.

10. Cherries:

Cherries, especially tart cherries, contain anthocyanins and other antioxidants. These compounds have been linked to reduced symptoms of gout and improved joint function.

11. Leafy Greens:

Leafy greens like spinach, kale, and Swiss chard are excellent sources of vitamins and minerals, including vitamin K and calcium, which are important for bone and joint health.

12. Low-Fat Dairy:

Low-fat dairy products, such as yogurt and milk, provide calcium and vitamin D, essential for strong bones and joint health.

Remember to maintain a balanced diet that incorporates a variety of these foods to reap their joint health benefits. While dietary changes can help alleviate joint pain, consult with a healthcare provider for a comprehensive approach to managing joint discomfort, which may include medications, exercise, and physical therapy.

7.2 Exercises for Joint Mobility

Maintaining joint mobility is essential for overall well-being, especially as we age. Stiff and inflexible joints can lead to discomfort and decreased mobility. Incorporating regular joint mobility exercises into your routine can help alleviate stiffness and improve your range of motion. Here are some excellent joint mobility exercises:

1. Neck Mobility Workouts:
Tilt your neck: Sit or stand with your back straight. Tilt your head slowly to one side, bringing your ear near your shoulder. Hold for a few seconds, then return to the neutral position. Repeat on the other side.

Neck Rotation: Gently turn your head to one side, as if looking over your shoulder. Hold for a few seconds, then return to the front. Repeat on the other side.

2. Shoulder Mobility Exercises:

Shoulder Rolls: Stand or sit with your arms at your sides. In a circular motion, slowly move your shoulders forward, then reverse and roll them backward. This exercise helps to reduce shoulder strain.

Stand with your feet shoulder-width apart for arm swings. Swing your arms forth and backward in a controlled motion, gradually expanding your range of motion.

3. Wrist and Hand Mobility Exercises:

Wrist Circles: Extend your arm in front of you, palm facing down. Slowly circle your wrist in one direction, then reverse the direction.

Finger Flexion and Extension: Spread your fingers apart as wide as possible, then make a fist. Repeat this motion to improve flexibility and circulation in the hands.

4. Hip Mobility Exercises:

Hip Circles: Stand with your hands on your hips. Circle your hips in a clockwise direction, then counterclockwise. This exercise can relieve hip tightness.

Hip Flexor Stretch: Step one foot forward and bend your knee while keeping your back leg straight. Lean forward slightly to feel a stretch in your hip flexors. Switch legs and repeat.

5. Knee Mobility Exercises:

Knee Extensions: Sit in a chair with your feet flat on the floor. Straighten one leg and hold for a few seconds, then bend it back to the starting position. Repeat with the other leg.

6. Ankle and Foot Mobility Exercises:

Ankle Circles: Sit with your feet flat on the floor. Lift one foot slightly and make slow circles with your ankle, first in one direction and then in the other. Repeat with the other foot.

Sit with your feet flat on the floor for toe flexion and extension. Curl your toes firmly and then spread them as far apart as you can.

7. Exercises for Spine Mobility:

Begin on your hands and knees for the Cat-Cow Stretch. Arch your back upward (as if you were a cat), then descend your spine while elevating your head (as if you were a cow). This motion should be repeated multiple times.

Torso twists are performed by sitting in a chair with your feet flat on the floor. Twist your torso to one side, using the back of the chair as support. Hold for a few seconds before twisting to the opposite side.

8. Full Body Mobility Exercises:

Tai Chi: This ancient Chinese practice combines gentle, flowing movements to promote joint mobility, balance, and relaxation. Consider taking Tai Chi classes to enhance overall flexibility.

Always perform these exercises in a controlled and pain-free manner. Start with gentle movements and gradually increase the range of motion as your joints become more flexible. If you have any existing medical conditions or joint problems, consult with a healthcare provider or physical therapist before starting a new exercise routine to ensure the exercises are safe and suitable for your needs.

8. Heart Health and Hypertension

8.1 Seniors and Heart Disease

Heart disease, including conditions such as coronary artery disease, heart failure, and arrhythmias, is a leading health concern for seniors. The risk of heart disease increases as we become older. Understanding the factors that contribute to heart disease in seniors and taking preventive measures is essential for maintaining heart health and overall well-being.

1. Aging and Heart Disease:

Several factors contribute to the increased risk of heart disease in seniors:

Atherosclerosis: Over time, the arteries can become narrowed and stiff due to the buildup of fatty deposits, leading to atherosclerosis. This restricts blood flow and can increase the risk of heart attacks and strokes.

Reduced Elasticity: Aging can cause changes in the heart's structure and function. The heart may become less efficient at pumping blood, and the arteries may lose their elasticity, affecting blood flow.

Chronic Health Conditions: Seniors often have chronic health conditions such as high blood pressure, diabetes, and high cholesterol, which are risk factors for heart disease.

2. Risk Factors for Heart Disease in Seniors:

High Blood Pressure: Hypertension is a major risk factor for heart disease. As we age, the likelihood of developing high blood pressure increases.

High Cholesterol: Elevated levels of cholesterol can lead to atherosclerosis, a common cause of heart disease. Seniors are more susceptible to high cholesterol.

Diabetes: Aging is associated with an increased risk of developing type 2 diabetes, which is a significant contributor to heart disease.

Physical Inactivity: Reduced physical activity in older adults can lead to weight gain, loss of muscle mass, and an increased risk of heart disease.

Smoking: Seniors who continue to smoke are at a higher risk of heart disease. Quitting smoking can lead to immediate and long-term benefits for heart health.

Obesity: Excess body weight, especially around the abdominal area, is a risk factor for heart disease. Maintaining a healthy weight is crucial for seniors.

Family History: A family history of heart disease can increase an individual's risk, especially as they age.

Diet: Poor dietary choices can contribute to heart disease. Seniors should focus on a heart-healthy diet rich in fruits, vegetables, whole grains, and lean proteins.

3. Preventive Measures:

Regular Check-ups: Seniors should have regular check-ups with healthcare providers to monitor blood pressure, cholesterol levels, and other heart disease risk factors.

Medication Management: If prescribed medications for conditions like high blood pressure or high cholesterol, it's essential to take them as directed.

Healthy Lifestyle: Adopting a heart-healthy lifestyle can help prevent heart disease. This includes regular physical activity, a balanced diet, and smoking cessation.

Stress Management: Chronic stress can contribute to heart disease. Seniors should practice stress-reduction techniques such as meditation, deep breathing, or yoga.

Medication Review: Seniors should periodically review their medications with their healthcare provider to ensure they are necessary and not causing side effects that could affect heart health.

Maintain Social Connections: Loneliness and isolation can contribute to heart disease. Seniors should stay socially engaged to support their mental and emotional well-being.

4. Heart Disease Symptoms in Seniors:

It's crucial for seniors to recognize the signs of heart disease, which may manifest differently than in younger individuals. Common symptoms can include chest pain, shortness of breath, fatigue, and irregular heart rhythms. If any of these symptoms are experienced, seeking prompt medical attention is essential.

9. Cognitive Function and Brain Health

9.1 Nutrients for a Sharp Mind

Maintaining a sharp mind is a key aspect of overall well-being, especially as we age. Nutrients play a crucial role in supporting brain health and cognitive function. Here are some essential nutrients that can help keep your mind sharp and functioning at its best:

1. Omega-3 Fatty Acids:

Omega-3 fatty acids, particularly docosahexaenoic acid (DHA) and eicosapentaenoic acid (EPA), are essential for brain health. They help build and maintain the structure of brain cells and promote communication between them. Fatty fish (salmon, mackerel, sardines), flaxseeds, chia seeds, and walnuts are good sources of omega-3s.

2. Antioxidants:

Antioxidants protect the brain from oxidative stress and inflammation, which can contribute to cognitive decline. Foods rich in antioxidants include colorful fruits and vegetables (berries, spinach, kale), green tea, and dark chocolate.

3. Vitamin E:

Vitamin E is a potent antioxidant that can help protect brain cells from oxidative damage. Vitamin E may be found in nuts, seeds, and vegetable oils.

4. B Vitamins:

B6, B9 (Folate), and B12: These vitamins support cognitive function and help reduce levels of homocysteine, an amino acid associated with cognitive decline. Good sources include leafy greens, legumes, fortified cereals, and lean meats.

5. Vitamin D:

Vitamin D plays a role in brain health, and low levels have been associated with cognitive decline. Sunlight exposure and vitamin D-rich foods like fatty fish, fortified dairy products, and eggs can help maintain optimal levels.

6. Iron:

Iron is essential for oxygen transport to the brain. Insufficient iron levels can lead to cognitive deficits and fatigue. Good sources of iron include lean meats, poultry, fish, and fortified cereals.

7. Zinc:

Zinc is necessary for the formation of new neurons and the transmission of signals between brain cells. It's found in foods like oysters, red meat, poultry, and whole grains.

8. Magnesium:

Magnesium is important for memory and learning. Foods like spinach, almonds, and black beans are excellent sources of magnesium.

9. Phosphatidylserine:

This phospholipid is a key component of cell membranes and is crucial for brain cell structure and function. It can be found in small amounts in foods like soy and organ meats or taken as a supplement.

10. Curcumin (Turmeric):

Curcumin, found in the spice turmeric, has anti-inflammatory and antioxidant properties. It may help improve memory and reduce the risk of neurodegenerative diseases.

11. Resveratrol:

Resveratrol, found in red grapes and red wine, has been associated with cognitive benefits and reduced risk of age-related memory decline.

12. Lutein and Zeaxanthin:

These carotenoids, primarily found in leafy greens and other colorful vegetables, have been linked to better cognitive function and memory.

13. Caffeine:

Moderate caffeine consumption, from sources like coffee and tea, can enhance alertness, concentration, and cognitive performance.

14. Water:

Hydration is essential for cognitive function. Even mild dehydration can affect cognitive abilities, so staying well-hydrated is crucial.

15. Choline:

Choline is important for the production of acetylcholine, a neurotransmitter that plays a role in memory and learning. Eggs, lean meats, and cruciferous vegetables are good sources of choline.

A balanced diet that incorporates a variety of nutrient-rich foods is the best way to support brain health and cognitive function. Additionally, staying physically active, getting adequate sleep, managing stress, and staying mentally engaged through activities like puzzles, reading, and learning new skills all contribute to a sharp mind. Consulting with a healthcare provider or registered dietitian can help you develop a personalized nutrition plan to support your cognitive well-being.

9.2 Brain-Boosting Activities

Engaging in brain-boosting activities is essential for maintaining cognitive function, mental agility, and overall brain health. Just like physical exercise keeps your body fit, mental exercises help keep your mind sharp. Here are various activities that can help enhance brain function and promote cognitive well-being:

1. Solve Puzzles:

Crossword Puzzles: These word puzzles challenge your vocabulary and memory.

Sudoku: Number puzzles like Sudoku improve logical reasoning and problem-solving skills.

2. Play Memory Games:

Memory Matching: Play games that involve matching cards or objects, enhancing your memory and concentration.

Lumosity and Brain-Training Apps: Numerous apps offer a variety of memory and cognitive training games designed to boost mental abilities.

3. Learn a New Language:

Studying a new language not only improves communication skills but also enhances cognitive functions like memory and multitasking.

4. Engage in Reading and Writing:

Reading: Regular reading stimulates the brain and enhances vocabulary and comprehension. Fiction, non-fiction, and newspapers all provide mental stimulation.

Writing: Keeping a journal, writing short stories, or blogging can improve creativity and cognitive abilities.

5. Stay Socially Active:

Engaging in conversations, attending social gatherings, and maintaining friendships are essential for mental well-being.

Participate in group activities like book clubs, game nights, or community events.

6. Pursue Hobbies:

Hobbies like painting, drawing, cooking, or playing a musical instrument offer creative and mental stimulation.

7. Practice Mindfulness and Meditation:

Mindfulness and meditation help reduce stress, improve focus, and enhance mental clarity.

8. Physical Exercise:

Regular physical activity enhances blood flow to the brain, promoting cognitive function and reducing the risk of cognitive decline.

9. Take Up Challenging Games:

Strategy-based games like chess, board games, or even video games can help improve problem-solving and critical thinking skills.

10. Educational Courses:

Enroll in classes or online courses to learn about topics that interest you. Lifelong learning is a great way to keep your mind active.

11. Brain-Teaser Books:

Solve brain teasers, riddles, and logic puzzles found in books or online resources.

12. Listen to Music:

Listening to classical music, in particular, has been associated with improved memory and focus.

13. Explore New Environments:

Traveling or simply exploring new places stimulates the brain by exposing it to novel experiences and environments.

14. Engage in Math Challenges:

Solve math problems or equations to boost your problem-solving skills and analytical thinking.

15. Gardening:

Gardening provides both physical and mental benefits, as it requires planning, organization, and attention to detail.

16. Volunteer:

Participating in volunteer work not only helps the community but also provides a sense of purpose and mental stimulation.

17. Play Brain-Training Video Games:

Certain video games are designed to improve cognitive skills such as memory, attention, and processing speed.

18. Mindful Eating:

Practicing mindful eating by savoring each bite and paying attention to flavors and textures can improve your attention and enjoyment of food.

19. Brain-Boosting Supplements:

Consult with a healthcare provider before considering supplements like fish oil, ginkgo biloba, or other nootropics.

Remember that the key to maintaining a sharp mind is to regularly engage in a variety of activities that challenge your brain. It's also essential to lead a healthy lifestyle by eating a balanced diet, staying physically active, getting sufficient sleep, and managing stress. By incorporating these activities into your daily routine, you can promote cognitive well-being and enjoy a mentally active and fulfilling life.

Chapter 5: Staying Active in Your Senior Years

10. The Importance of Senior Fitness

10.1 Age-Appropriate Exercises

Staying physically active as a senior is crucial for maintaining good health, mobility, and overall quality of life. Age-appropriate exercises are tailored to the unique needs and abilities of older adults. These exercises can help improve strength, flexibility, balance, and cardiovascular health, while also reducing the risk of falls and chronic health conditions. Here are some age-appropriate exercises for seniors:

1. Walking:

Walking is a simple and effective exercise that can be tailored to individual fitness levels. It's low-impact, gentle on the joints, and can be done both indoors and outside. Seniors can start with short walks and gradually increase the duration as they become more comfortable.

2. Strength Training:

Strength training exercises help seniors maintain muscle mass and bone density. Light resistance exercises using resistance bands, hand weights, or bodyweight can be beneficial. Common strength exercises for seniors include:

Leg lifts are a great way to strengthen your lower body.
Push-ups against a wall to develop the upper body.
Leg extensions while seated to target leg muscles.
Light hand weights for bicep curls.

3. Chair Exercises:

Chair exercises are ideal for seniors with mobility limitations. They can be performed while sitting in a sturdy chair. Examples include seated leg lifts, seated marches, and seated side leg lifts.

4. Balance Exercises:

Balance exercises are important for preventing falls, a common concern for seniors. Simple balance exercises include:

Standing on one leg for a few seconds, then switching to the other leg.

Heel-to-toe walking to improve balance and coordination.

Balancing on one foot while holding onto a stable surface for support.

5. Stretching and Flexibility:

Stretching exercises help maintain flexibility and range of motion. Seniors can perform gentle stretches to improve flexibility in major muscle groups. Yoga and Tai Chi are also excellent options for flexibility and balance.

6. Water Aerobics:

Water aerobics is a low-impact exercise that reduces stress on the joints. Seniors can participate in group classes or perform water exercises in a pool. Water resistance provides a gentle workout for both cardiovascular health and strength.

7. Cycling:

Cycling, either on a stationary bike or a regular bicycle, is a great way to improve cardiovascular health while being gentle on the joints.

8. Dancing:

Dancing can be a fun and social way to stay active. There are many dance styles suitable for seniors, such as ballroom dancing, line dancing, or Zumba.

9. Mind-Body Exercises:

Mind-body exercises like Tai Chi and Qi Gong offer a combination of movement and meditation. They enhance balance, flexibility, and mental well-being.

10. Low-Impact Aerobics:

Low-impact aerobic classes designed for seniors offer a full-body workout without the jarring impact of high-impact exercises.

Seniors should contact a healthcare physician before beginning any fitness program to verify that the exercises they choose are safe and appropriate for their specific health needs. It's important to start slowly, listen to your body, and gradually increase the intensity and duration of your workouts. Staying active and engaged in age-appropriate exercises can greatly improve the quality of life for seniors, promoting independence and vitality as they age.

10.2 Staying Active at Home

For seniors, staying active at home is essential for maintaining physical health, mental well-being, and independence. Regular exercise can improve mobility, reduce the risk of chronic conditions, and enhance overall quality of life. Here are some tips and exercises tailored to seniors for staying active at home:

1. Consult with a Healthcare Provider:

Before starting any new fitness plan, talk to your doctor, especially if you have any underlying medical concerns or haven't been active in a long time. They can provide guidance and ensure your chosen exercises are safe for your individual health needs.

2. Warm-Up and Cool Down:

Always start with a warm-up to prepare your muscles and joints for exercise, and finish with a cool-down to gradually reduce your heart rate and prevent muscle stiffness.

3. Aerobic Exercise:

Aerobic exercises promote cardiovascular health and help maintain stamina. Suitable activities for seniors at home include:

Walking: Indoors or in your garden, walking is a low-impact exercise that can be adapted to your fitness level.

Chair Exercises: Seated leg lifts, seated marches, and seated side leg lifts can provide a cardiovascular workout while sitting in a sturdy chair.

Dancing: Put on your favorite music and have a dance session. It's an enjoyable way to get your heart rate up.

4. Strength Training:

Strength exercises are crucial for maintaining muscle mass and bone density. Light resistance exercises using resistance bands, hand weights, or body weight can be beneficial. Common strength exercises for seniors include:

Leg raises to strengthen the lower body.

Wall push-ups to work the upper body.

Bicep curls with light hand weights.

Seated leg extensions to target leg muscles.

5. Balance Exercises:

Balance exercises are important for preventing falls, a common concern for seniors. Simple balance exercises include:

Standing on one leg for a few seconds, then switching to the other leg.

Heel-to-toe walking to improve balance and coordination.

Balancing on one foot while holding onto a stable surface for support.

6. Flexibility and Stretching:

Stretching exercises help maintain flexibility and range of motion. Perform gentle stretches to improve flexibility in major muscle groups. Yoga and Tai Chi are also excellent options for flexibility and balance.

7. Breathing and Relaxation:

Incorporate deep breathing exercises and relaxation techniques to reduce stress and enhance mental well-being. This can include guided breathing exercises and meditation.

8. Stay Hydrated:

Proper hydration is crucial for overall health and exercise performance. Drink plenty of water before, during, and after your workouts.

9. Household Activities:

Everyday household activities like vacuuming, sweeping, or gardening can provide physical activity and contribute to your daily exercise routine.

10. Stay Connected:

Participate in virtual fitness classes or join online fitness communities. This adds a social component to your workouts and provides motivation.

11. Set Goals:

Set achievable fitness goals for yourself. This can help you stay motivated and track your progress.

12. Safety First:

Make sure your exercise area is well-lit and free from hazards like rugs or cords that can cause tripping. Have a phone nearby in case of emergencies.

13. Rest and Recovery:

Listen to your body and give it time to rest and recover between workouts, especially if you experience any discomfort or pain.

Staying active at home for seniors is not only possible but highly beneficial. Regular physical activity can improve your quality of life, maintain independence, and promote overall health and well-being. By incorporating age-appropriate exercises and following safety guidelines, you can enjoy a healthier and more active lifestyle, even within the confines of your home.

Chapter 6: Monitoring Progress and Making Adjustments

11. Tracking Your Senior Metabolic Confusion Journey

11.1 Identifying Plateaus

Exercise plateaus can be frustrating, but they are a common part of any fitness journey, regardless of age. For seniors, recognizing and overcoming plateaus is essential to continue making progress and maintain a healthy and active lifestyle. Here's how to identify exercise plateaus and strategies for overcoming them:

Identifying Exercise Plateaus:

Lack of Progress: One clear sign of a plateau is a significant lack of progress in your fitness routine. If you've been doing the same exercises at the same intensity for an extended period and don't notice any improvements, it's time to reassess.

Boredom: Boredom or a lack of motivation can be another indication that you've hit a plateau. If you find your workouts monotonous or no longer enjoyable, it's a sign that you might need a change.

Injuries and Aches: If you experience more aches, pains, or injuries during your workouts, it might be due to overuse of certain exercises. This can signal a plateau.

Stagnant Strength: If your strength levels have plateaued, and you're unable to lift heavier weights or perform more repetitions, it's time to evaluate your routine.

Overcoming Exercise Plateaus:

Change Your Routine: One of the most effective ways to break a plateau is to change your exercise routine. Try different exercises, variations, or introduce new equipment or techniques.

Increase Intensity: Gradually increase the intensity of your workouts. This might mean lifting heavier weights, doing more reps, or adding interval training to your cardiovascular routine.

Opt for Cross-Training: Incorporate cross-training into your fitness regimen. Engage in a variety of activities such as strength training, cardio, flexibility, and balance exercises. Cross-training prevents overuse injuries and keeps your body challenged.

Set New Goals: Set precise and attainable goals. This could be related to strength, endurance, flexibility, or any other aspect of your fitness. Having clear goals will provide motivation and a sense of purpose.

Monitor Nutrition: Ensure your diet supports your fitness goals. Eating a balanced diet that includes sufficient protein, healthy fats, and carbohydrates is vital for recovery and progress.

Recovery and Rest: Don't underestimate the importance of rest and recovery. Overtraining can lead to plateaus and injuries. Make sure you allow your body to recover properly between workouts.

Consult a Professional: If you're unsure how to overcome a plateau or have concerns about your fitness routine, consider consulting a fitness professional or physical therapist who can provide expert guidance.

Stay Consistent: Consistency is key to making long-term progress. Ensure you maintain a regular exercise routine, even when facing plateaus.

Mental Approach: Keep in mind that fitness is a journey with ups and downs.

appreciate tiny Wins: Recognize and appreciate tiny victories along the road. Recognizing these successes can boost your motivation and help you stay committed.

As a senior, it's essential to be patient with yourself and listen to your body. You may progress at a slower pace, but consistent effort and the right strategies can help you break through plateaus and continue to improve your fitness and overall well-being.

Chapter 7: A Lifetime of Senior Health

12. Aging Gracefully with Metabolic Confusion

12.1 Long-Term Health Benefits

As seniors embrace healthy lifestyles, they can reap numerous long-term health benefits that contribute to a fulfilling and active aging process. By adopting a combination of regular exercise, balanced nutrition, and other positive habits, seniors can experience the following long-term health advantages:

1. Enhanced Cardiovascular Health:

Reduced Risk of Heart Disease: Regular exercise and a heart-healthy diet help manage blood pressure, cholesterol levels, and reduce the risk of heart disease.

Stronger Heart: Exercise improves cardiac efficiency, which can lead to a lower risk of heart failure.

2. Weight Management:

Weight Control: Healthy eating and regular physical activity help seniors maintain a healthy weight, reducing the risk of obesity-related conditions.

Reduced Risk of Obesity: Staying active and following a balanced diet are essential for preventing and managing obesity.

3. Cognitive Health:

Reduced Risk of Cognitive Decline: Engaging in mentally stimulating activities, such as puzzles and learning, can support cognitive function and reduce the risk of cognitive decline.
4. Bone Health:

Preserved Bone Density: Weight-bearing exercises like walking and strength training help maintain bone density, reducing the risk of osteoporosis.

5. Diabetes Management:

Improved Blood Sugar Control: Exercise and a balanced diet assist in regulating blood sugar levels, which can be valuable for managing diabetes.
6. Respiratory Health:

Enhanced Lung Function: Regular physical activity supports lung function and overall respiratory health.
7. Cancer Prevention:

Reduced Risk of Certain Cancers: A healthy lifestyle, including regular exercise, is associated with a reduced risk of specific cancers, such as breast, colon, and lung cancer.
8. Joint Health:

Stronger Joints: Appropriate exercise can strengthen muscles around the joints, reducing the risk of joint pain and arthritis.
9. Sleep Quality:

Improved Sleep: Regular physical activity can enhance sleep quality and alleviate insomnia.

10. Emotional Well-Being:

Stress Reduction: Exercise contributes to stress reduction and relaxation, leading to improved emotional well-being.

Better Mood: Physical activity stimulates the release of endorphins, which can improve mood and promote a positive outlook.

11. Social Engagement:

Community and Social Connections: Participating in group activities or fitness classes fosters social connections and emotional well-being.
12. Quality of Life:

Enhanced Quality of Life: Seniors who embrace a healthy lifestyle enjoy a higher quality of life, with greater mobility and a reduced risk of chronic diseases.
13. Independence in Aging:

Maintained Independence: Staying active and healthy can help seniors maintain their independence and reduce the risk of disability in aging.

14. Better Immune Response:

Stronger Immune Response: Regular exercise can enhance the immune system's ability to fight off infections, keeping seniors healthier and more resilient.
15. Lifelong Learning:

Cognitive Enrichment: Continuing to learn and engage in mentally stimulating activities contributes to cognitive enrichment and long-term brain health.
16. Healthy Relationships:

Positive Social Connections: Maintaining healthy relationships and social engagement with family, friends, and the community contributes to a fulfilling and long life.

It's never too late for seniors to adopt a healthier lifestyle and enjoy the long-term health benefits it brings. These rewards are cumulative and increase with continued commitment to health and well-being. By embracing a balanced diet, regular exercise, and other healthy habits, seniors can age gracefully while enjoying a more fulfilling and active retirement.

12.2 Tips for Maintaining Your Health

For seniors, maintaining health is a valuable pursuit that can lead to a more active, enjoyable, and fulfilling life. Here are some essential tips to help seniors preserve their well-being and age gracefully:

1. Stay Active:

Regular physical activity is essential for seniors. Engage in exercises that are appropriate for your age and fitness level. Focus on activities that promote strength, flexibility, and balance.

2. Nutrient-Rich Diet:

Maintain a nutritious diet rich in fruits, vegetables, whole grains, lean proteins, and healthy fats. Proper nutrition is key to overall health.

3. Regular Health Checkups:

Visit your healthcare provider for regular checkups and screenings. These can help detect and manage health issues in their early stages.

4. Mental Health Matters:

Prioritize your mental health. Practice stress management, engage in activities that promote relaxation, and seek support for emotional concerns.

5. Quality Sleep:

Make an effort to obtain 7-9 hours of decent sleep every night. Establish a consistent sleep schedule and create a calming bedtime routine.

6. Stay Hydrated:

Drinking enough water is crucial. Dehydration can have adverse effects on health, so make an effort to stay well-hydrated.

7. Avoid Smoking and Limit Alcohol:

If you smoke, consider quitting, and limit alcohol consumption to reduce health risks.

8. Sun Protection:

Protect your skin from the sun by wearing sunscreen and appropriate clothing. Avoid excessive sun exposure to lower the risk of skin cancer.

9. Weight Management:

Maintaining a healthy weight is vital for overall health. Consult a healthcare provider or nutritionist if you need assistance with weight management.

10. Manage Stress:

Use relaxation techniques, mindfulness, meditation, or hobbies you enjoy to manage stress effectively. Chronic stress can have negative impacts on health.

11. Stay Social:

Nurture your social connections with family and friends. Social engagement enhances emotional well-being and combats feelings of loneliness.

12. Health Screenings and Immunizations:

Adhere to recommended health screening guidelines and stay up-to-date with vaccinations to protect against diseases and conditions.

13. Mindful Eating:

Practice mindful eating by savoring your meals and paying attention to your body's hunger and fullness cues. Avoid overeating or mindless eating.

14. Safety First:

Prevent falls and accidents by making your home safer. Install handrails, non-slip surfaces, and adequate lighting.

15. Lifelong Learning:

Stimulate your mind through continuous learning and mental challenges. Engaging in new experiences and hobbies can promote cognitive health.

16. Volunteer and Give Back:

Participating in volunteer work and helping others can provide a sense of purpose and fulfillment, contributing to your well-being.

17. Dental Health:

Oral health is vital. Visit the dentist for regular checkups and maintain good oral hygiene practices.

18. Regular Medication Management:

If you're on medications, ensure that you take them as prescribed and communicate with your healthcare provider about any concerns or side effects.

19. Listen to Your Body:

Take note of any unexpected symptoms or pain. Promptly seek medical advice or assistance when needed.

20. Embrace Technology:

Don't be afraid to use technology to help manage your health, such as smartphone apps for medication reminders or virtual doctor visits.

Conclusion

In the pages of this book, we've explored the transformative power of the Metabolic Confusion Diet tailored specifically for seniors. It's a journey that has taken us through the intricacies of metabolic processes, the unique dietary needs of aging bodies, and the science behind this groundbreaking approach to health and well-being. As we conclude, let's reflect on the key takeaways and the incredible potential that this diet offers to seniors seeking to improve their quality of life.

The Metabolic Confusion Diet for Seniors is not just a diet; it's a way of life designed to optimize health and vitality. It recognizes that seniors have distinct nutritional requirements, and it adapts to these needs, offering a tailored approach that can help address age-related challenges.

As we've discovered, the science of metabolic confusion is rooted in the notion that regularly changing your dietary patterns keeps your metabolism agile and responsive. This approach can lead to numerous benefits, including weight management, improved energy levels, better cognitive function, enhanced cardiovascular health, and a reduced risk of chronic diseases.

Furthermore, the Metabolic Confusion Diet acknowledges that dietary restrictions, digestive issues, and other health concerns are common among seniors. It provides strategies to navigate these challenges while still reaping the rewards of the diet.

Hydration, meal timing, and daily meal structure have all been explored in detail, emphasizing their significance in optimizing the diet's effectiveness. The diet offers a flexible approach to fit into the rhythms of seniors' lives, making it sustainable and practical.

We've also delved into the diverse food choices available to seniors, ensuring that the diet remains enjoyable and diverse. Sample meal plans have provided practical guidance, allowing for ease of implementation. Additionally, recommendations for alleviating joint pain and exercises to promote joint mobility have been presented, recognizing the importance of physical health in senior years.

The Metabolic Confusion Diet for Seniors is more than just a dietary regimen; it's a holistic approach that recognizes the interconnectedness of physical and mental well-being. We've discussed the importance of mental clarity and brain-boosting activities, as well as the value of age-appropriate exercises and heart disease prevention.

The book has touched on the significance of nutrients for a sharp mind, age-appropriate exercises, and brain-boosting activities, underlining the idea that a healthy mind is as vital as a healthy body.

In conclusion, the Metabolic Confusion Diet for Seniors offers a comprehensive strategy for seniors to enhance their health and vitality. It's a diet that celebrates the wisdom and experience that come with age, and it recognizes that growing older doesn't mean sacrificing a vibrant and active life. With the guidance provided in this book, seniors have the tools to take charge of their health and embrace the journey toward a healthier, happier, and more fulfilling life.

It's important to remember that adopting any new diet or lifestyle change should be done in consultation with a healthcare provider to ensure that it aligns with your individual health needs. Your healthcare provider can offer personalized guidance and support as you embark on this exciting journey towards better health.

With the knowledge and strategies outlined in this book, seniors have the opportunity to savor the benefits of the Metabolic Confusion Diet, reinvigorate their lives, and savor the golden years with boundless energy and vitality. Here's to your health, happiness, and a bright future ahead!